Fit and Flavorful

2024 Diet Dishes for a Healthier You

Dr. John T. Grover

1

COPYRIGHT

DEDICATION

Dedicated to all those on a journey to nourish their bodies and delight their palates. May the pages of 'Fit and Flavorful' inspire you to embrace the harmonious blend of health and taste, and empower you to savor every moment of your wellness quest. This book is dedicated to you, with gratitude for choosing to prioritize your well-being and enjoyment.

Author Bio

Dr. John T. Grover is a distinguished author whose expertise transcends boundaries, blending his profound knowledge in the field of expertise with a passion for storytelling. With a wealth of experience, he navigates the complexities of specific subjects with a unique narrative flair, making his works both intellectually stimulating and accessible to a diverse audience. Driven by a relentless curiosity, he has authored numerous insightful publications, earning him recognition as a thought leader in relevant industry. His commitment to excellence in both academia and literature makes Dr. Grover a compelling voice in the literary landscape.

Table of contents

INTRODUCTION

Welcome to a Healthier You

where we begin out on a journey to vitality and

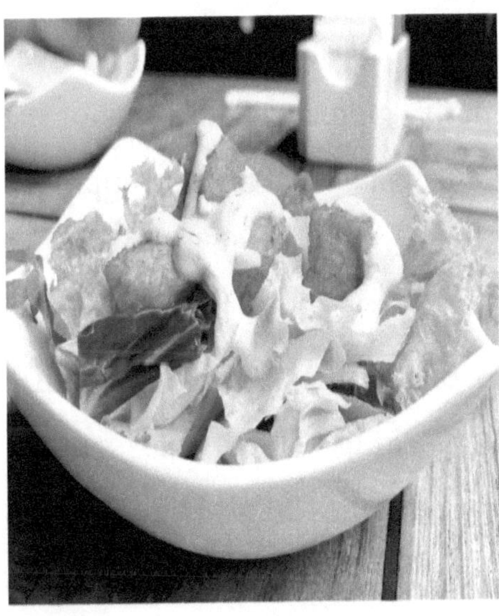

total well-being. This platform functions as your compass in a world where establishing a healthy lifestyle is becoming more and more crucial. It provides you with evidence-based techniques, intelligent counsel, and strong strategies. "Welcome to a Healthier You" is your trusted companion in obtaining long-term health and happiness, regardless of your goals—whether they are to enhance your mental and emotional health, establish harmonious relationships with others, or raise your physical fitness. Come along as we take a step at a time as we explore the roads leading to a complete and fulfilled living.

In order to properly appreciate the ideas of the 2024 Diet, one must analyze a holistic approach for nutrition and general health that has a focus on sustainable and scientifically validated practices. Based on the most current scientific discoveries and taking into consideration personal preferences, the 2024 Diet stresses several fundamental tenets:

1. Whole Foods Emphasis: Eating whole, less processed foods is the cornerstone of the 2024 Diet. Fruits, vegetables, whole grains, lean meats, and healthy fats are a few of them.

People may reduce intake of added sugars, processed carbs, and toxic fats while nourishing their bodies with critical vitamins, minerals, and antioxidants by making these nutrient-dense meals a priority.

2. Balanced Macronutrients: For maximum health, the distribution of macronutrients fats, proteins, and carbohydrates must be balanced. The 2024 Diet emphasizes a well-rounded approach, emphasizing lean proteins like fish, poultry, and plant-based alternatives, complex carbohydrates from whole grains and legumes, and healthy fats from nuts, seeds, avocados, and olive oil.

3. Portion Control and Mindful Eating: Two crucial components of the 2024 Diet are being conscious of portion proportions and participating in mindful eating. People may strengthen their relationship with food, prevent overindulging, and have a greater appreciation for the flavors and textures of their food by learning to understand their hunger and fullness signals.

4. Hydration: Drinking adequate water is vital for overall health and wellness in general. Drinking water throughout the day is vital to keeping sufficient hydration, according to the 2024 Diet. Water, herbal teas, and other hydrating fluids are preferable alternatives for maintaining hydration goals and ensuring normal body function when sugary beverages are drunk in moderation.

5. Flexibility and Individualization: The 2024 Diet emphasizes the significance of flexibility and individualization while proposing broad parameters for a healthy diet. The 2024 Diet lets individuals tailor their food choices dependent on their specific nutritional needs, preferences, and ambitions. Flexibility is necessary for long-term adherence and success, whether it is for changing to cultural or lifestyle standards, fulfilling dietary limitations, or addressing food sensitivities.

6.Physical activity: Consistent physical exercise is vital for maintaining overall health and managing weight, in addition to healthy food. The 2024 Diet lays a high focus on the benefits of incorporating physical activity into regular activities, whether via scheduled exercises, outdoor hobbies, or simply creating more time for movement in general.

CHAPTER ONE

Breakfast Boosters

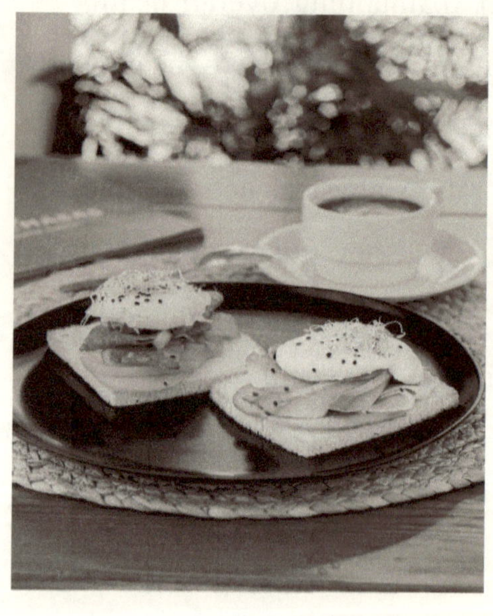

For good reason, breakfast is frequently described as the most crucial meal of the day. It wakes up your metabolism, replenishes your energy stores, and provides the framework for the remainder of your day's dietary choices. Consider adding breakfast boosters—nutrient-rich foods and strategies that increase the nutritional content and overall health advantages of your morning meal—to maximize its benefits. The following breakfast-boosting recommendations will help you launch your morning routine:

1. Protein Power: Eating a breakfast heavy in protein may help you feel full and satisfied until your next meal. Think about items like smoked salmon, eggs, cottage cheese, Greek yogurt, and tofu. For a fast protein boost, you may also throw in a scoop of protein powder to smoothies or porridge.

2. Fiber Friends: Fiber increases fullness, reduces blood sugar, and helps with digestion. Start your day with foods rich in fiber, such as nuts and seeds (almonds, chia seeds, and flaxseeds), fruits (bananas, apples, and berries), vegetables (spinach, avocado, and bell peppers), and whole grains (oats, quinoa, and whole wheat bread).

3. Healthy Fats: Including healthy fats in your breakfast may assist sustain brain function and offer you long-lasting energy. Tasty alternatives to integrate healthy fats into your morning meal include avocado slices on whole grain toast, a dab of nut butter in your smoothie or oatmeal, or a sprinkle of seeds over your yogurt.

4. Colorful Produce: To maximize your intake of vitamins, minerals, and antioxidants, aim to consume a variety of colorful fruits and vegetables for breakfast. Leafy greens, tomatoes, kiwi, citrus fruits, and berries are all fantastic selections that boost the flavor and nutritional value of your diet.

5.Hydration Aids: Remember to remain hydrated first thing in the morning! Drinking a glass of water or herbal tea first thing in the morning can aid your body recover moisture from the previous night's sleep and speed up your metabolism. For extra flavor, try adding bits of citrus fruit, cucumber, or mint to your water.

6.Meal Planning and Prep: Make your breakfast a success by arranging and preparing it ahead of time. Breakfast burritos, egg muffins, and overnight oats are a few examples of foods that may be batch prepared to save time in the morning rush and assure a nutritious breakfast.

7. Mindful Eating: Give your breakfast some thought and savor it, concentrating on the flavors, textures, and sensations of every bite. You may increase digestion and satisfaction by eating slowly and attentively, which will make you feel more filled and active all day.

Smoothies in the morning are a pleasant and practical way to start your day off with a consistent energy boost and a burst of nutrients. These smoothies, which are full with fruits, veggies, protein, and healthy fats, deliver your body a well-balanced blend of macronutrients to support maximum health. Here's how to develop informative information about revitalizing smoothies for breakfast:

Energizing Morning Smoothies

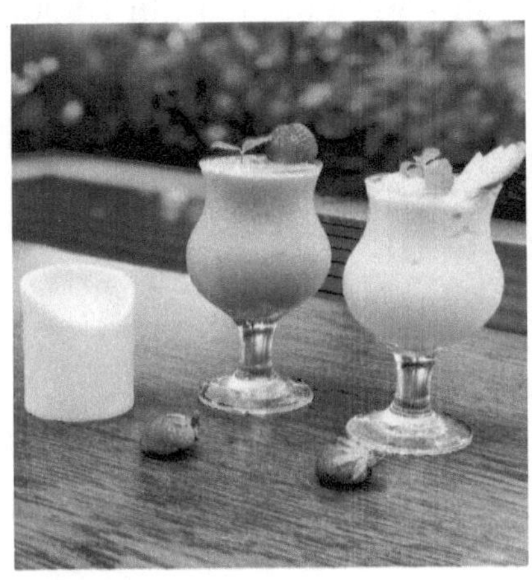

1.High-Nutrient Components: Stress the significance of integrating nutrient-dense foods like leafy greens (kale, spinach), fruits (mango, banana, and berries), vegetables (carrots, cucumber), and superfoods (chia seeds, flaxseeds, and spirulina) into your smoothies. These components fuel your body and improve overall well-being by delivering vitamins, minerals, antioxidants, and fiber.

2. Protein Power: Adding protein to your morning smoothie helps regulate blood sugar levels, supports muscle building and repair, and keeps you feeling full and delighted until your next meal. To improve the protein content of your smoothie, add protein sources like nut butter, Greek yogurt, protein powder (whey, pea, hemp), or silken tofu.

3. Balanced Flavor Profiles: To keep your morning smoothies interesting and delightful, consider experimenting with varied flavor combinations. Try balancing savory vegetables and sweet fruits, adding a dash of citrus or spice for some brightness, or adding herbs like basil or mint for a cool touch. Promote creativity and customisation in line with individual preferences.

4.Tips and Tricks for Preparation: Give suggestions on how to create smoothies fast and simply. Some ideas are to chop items ahead of time, use frozen fruits and veggies for ease, and buy a good blender for smooth, creamy results. Give advice on how to freeze leftover smoothie portions or make smoothie packs in bulk for quick and simple breakfast alternatives on hectic mornings.

5.Hydration and Refreshment: Include hydrating components in your smoothies, such as coconut water, cucumber, or fruits high in the amount of water it contains, to highlight the need of maintaining proper hydration first thing in the morning. These components help you feel refreshed and energetic throughout the day by adding a refreshing aspect to your morning routine and aiding with hydration.

6.thoughtful Consumption: Promote the thoughtful consuming smoothies by focusing on emotions of nutrition and pleasure as well as taking the time to taste each drink and appreciate the flavors and textures. Remind readers to pay attention to their bodies and modify the components in smoothies according to their degree of hunger, preferred diets, and unique nutritional requirements.

Protein-Packed Breakfast Wrap

Breakfast wraps loaded with protein are a tasty

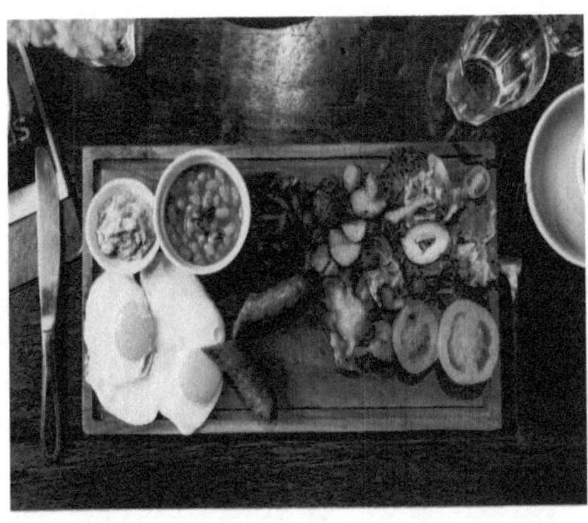

and filling way to get your day started with a healthy boost. These wraps provide a handy, portable choice that's loaded with protein to keep you feeling full and energized—perfect for refueling after a workout or fueling up before a hectic morning. Here's how to write an engaging article on breakfast wraps that are high in protein:

Start by emphasizing the value of protein in the morning with .

1.The Power of Protein. Protein is a crucial part of a healthy breakfast since it supports muscle development and repair, blood sugar regulation, and satiety.

2.Wrap Base Options: Offer a variety of wrap bases to use as the starting point for your breakfast wraps that are loaded with protein. The basis of your components is made up of whole grain tortillas, spinach or kale wraps, or low-carb substitutes like collard greens or lettuce leaves. All of these options are high in fiber and nutrients.

3. **Protein, in particular, Fillings**: Presenting a range of fillings that are high in protein that you may use in your breakfast wraps. Greek yogurt, egg whites, tofu, smoked salmon, turkey or chicken sausage, black beans, or chickpeas are some of the options. Urge readers to adjust the components to suit their nutritional needs and dietary choices.

4. Vegetable Boost: Including veggies in your breakfast wraps gives them taste and texture as well as important minerals, vitamins, and antioxidants. For extra nutrients and color, add alternatives like sautéed spinach, bell peppers, onions, mushrooms, tomatoes, avocado slices, or shredded carrots.

5. Flavor Enhancers: Use seasonings like herbs, spices, and sauces to bring out the flavor of your protein-rich breakfast wraps. For an added kick, add a dollop of pesto or hummus, a drizzle of balsamic glaze or sriracha mayo, a sprinkle of fresh herbs like cilantro or parsley, and a dash of spicy sauce or salsa.

6. Meal Prep Tips: Share meal prep ideas to help you save time on hectic mornings by making protein-rich breakfast wraps ahead of time. Make items like grilled chicken or scrambled eggs in advance, put together the wraps the night before, or wrap each one separately and store it in the freezer or refrigerator for easy grab-and-go meals.

7.Customization and Adaptability: Inspire readers to personalize their protein-rich breakfast wraps according to their dietary requirements, dietary inclinations, or dietary restrictions. To suit a range of dietary requirements and preferences, include ideas for low-carb, gluten-free, or vegetarian solutions.

8.Portion Control and Balance: When putting together their breakfast wraps, readers should remember to exercise portion control and aim for balance. Aim for a combination of healthy fats, carbs, and protein. Pay attention to portion proportions so that the wrap doesn't include too many calories or macros.

CHAPTER TWO

Lively Lunches

Lunch is more than simply a time to recharge around noon; it's a chance to take a breather,

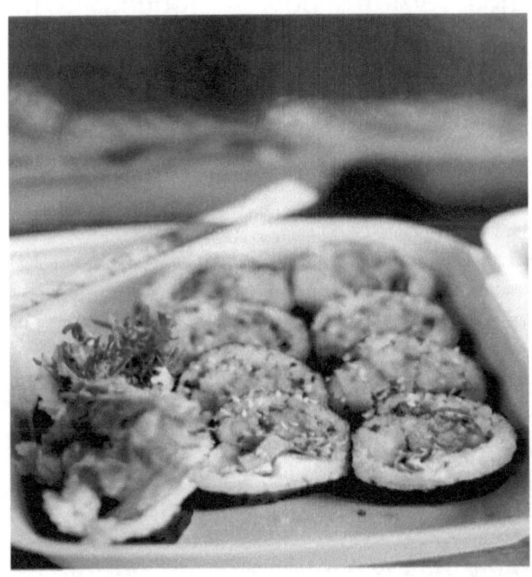

relax, and enjoy a fulfilling meal that fulfills both the body and the soul. Whether you're dining with loved ones, having a lonely lunch without a break, or meeting with colleagues, these options might help you spice up your midday meals:

1. Colorful Creations: Add a selection of brilliant fruits, veggies, and other colorful foods to your lunch to make it both visually beautiful and nutrient-rich. Imagine salads loaded with mixed greens and savory dressing, or rainbow-shaped grain bowls topped with roasted veggies, cherry tomatoes, bell peppers, carrots, and sliced avocado.

2. Global tastes: Create a midday supper that takes you on a gourmet journey of the globe by utilizing tastes and ingredients from various cultures. Try the Thai-inspired noodle salad with peanut sauce, the Mexican-inspired grain bowl with black beans, salsa, and guacamole on top, or the Mediterranean wrap with hummus, olives, and grilled veggies.

3. Protein Power: To retain your energy and satisfaction late into the afternoon, make sure you eat an adequate quantity of protein throughout lunch. Incorporate lean protein sources like grilled chicken, lentils, quinoa, beans, and tofu into your meals. Try adding nuts, seeds, or a tiny bit of cheese for some extra taste and nutrients.

4. Creative Combos: Mix and mix various food categories and textures to generate fascinating and substantial lunchtime meals. Mix meals high in protein with nutritious grains, healthy fats, and lots of veggies to prepare a well-balanced lunch that will fill you up and give you energy for the entire day.

5. Happiness Made at Home: Prepare your own lunches whenever feasible. Not only will you avoid waste and save money, but you will also have control over the tastes and ingredients. Batch prepare components like grains, roasted veggies, and protein at the beginning of the week to speed up lunchtime assembling.

6. Mindful Moments: Take advantage of your lunch break by practicing mindfulness and relishing your meal. Put your electronics aside, rise up from your desk, and concentrate on the sensations, tastes, and textures of every mouthful. Eating attentively and slowly may boost enjoyment and digestion while also lowering stress and increasing overall wellbeing.

7. Social ties: If you have the chance, have lunch with them to establish relationships and social connections. Eating lunch with friends, family, or colleagues may improve the overall meal experience by promoting a feeling of joy and camaraderie.

8. On-the-Go Options: On busy days when you're pushed for time, prepare sandwiches that are easy to carry and that you can eat anywhere. Prepare a huge cereal bowl in a reusable container, pack a salad in a mason jar, or construct a wrap or sandwich in preparation for a healthy on-the-go lunch.

Crisp, fresh salads are not only tasty and gratifying, but they're also a terrific way to add a range of foods rich in nutrients into your diet. Whether you eat these salads as a colorful main course, a light lunch, or a chilled side dish, they will excite your palate and fuel your health. This is how to make intriguing articles about crisp, fresh salads:

Fresh and Crunchy Salads

Nourishing Grain Bowls

Fresh and Crunchy Salads

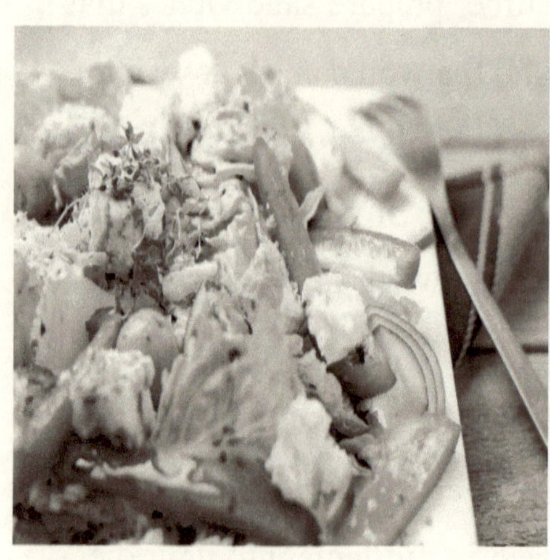

1. Vibrant components: Emphasize how vital it is to incorporate a variety of colorful foods to your salads to increase their taste and nutritional worth. Add a variety of fresh produce, including bell peppers, carrots, radishes, tomatoes, cucumbers, and leafy greens, as well as some sweet fruits and vegetables like apples, oranges, or berries.

2. Crunchy Texture: Emphasize how vital it is to integrate crunchy ingredients into your salads to improve their texture and offer a pleasing crunch. Add ingredients such as chopped nuts (almonds, walnuts, pecans), seeds (pumpkin, sunflower), crispy croutons, or crunchy vegetables (celery, jicama, water chestnuts) for added visual appeal and textural contrast.

3. Protein Boost: Include high-protein foods in your salads to make them more substantial and delicious. Options include grilled chicken or tofu, chopped cheese, quinoa, edamame, hard-boiled eggs, and other foods. Protein helps you feel satiated and full while boosting muscle development and repair.

4. Healthy Fats: Don't forget to incorporate healthy fats to your salads to improve satiety and give a source of continuous energy. Add toppings like avocado slices, olives, nuts, seeds, or a drizzle of olive oil to increase taste and texture while also providing a portion of heart-healthy fats.

5.Delicious Dressings: A well-crafted dressing transforms a plain salad into a memorable dinner. Try making your own dressings by experimenting with items like mustard, citrus juice, vinegar, olive oil, herbs, and spices to create taste combinations that compliment the other elements in your salad. Encourage readers to prepare their own dressings so they may keep in command of the ingredients and adjust the flavors to fit their preferences.

6. Seasonal Variations: To represent the shifting of the seasons, add seasonal items to your salads. Use in-season, fresh, ripe ingredients for optimum taste and nutrition. Consider springtime food like asparagus, strawberries, and delicate greens; midsummer produce like tomatoes, maize, and peaches; autumn produce like apples, squash, and Brussels sprouts; and winters stuff like citrus fruits, kale, and root vegetables.

7. Inventive Mixtures: Encourage creativity and experimenting with salad ingredients and tastes. Readers are asked to venture outside the box and explore various ingredients, textures, and taste combinations to keep their salads exciting and fresh.

Nourishing Grain Bowls

Nutritious grain bowls are a delightful and varied way to enjoy a well-balanced meal full of taste, texture, and nutrients. A foundation of wholesome grains, an array of veggies, protein-rich toppings, and delightful sauces or dressings make up

grain bowls, which are adaptable, quick to cook, and excellent for any time of day. Here's how to make fascinating articles about grain bowls that are healthy:

1. Wholesome Base: Let me start by underlining how crucial it is to base your grain bowl with whole grains. Brown rice, quinoa, farro, barley, and bulgur are among the grains that are rich in fiber, vitamins, minerals, and long-lasting energy to keep you feeling content and full.

2.Abundant veggies: Use a variety of colorful veggies to add texture, taste, and nutrition to your grain bowl. Add both cooked and fresh veggies, such roasted sweet potatoes, sautéed bell peppers, sliced cucumbers, steamed broccoli, and shredded carrots, for a colorful and nutrient-dense blend.

3. Protein Powerhouses: Top your grain bowl with high-protein toppings to boost its fillingness and delight. Among the options are edamame, black beans, lentils, chickpeas, tofu, and tempeh. Strike a balance between plant- and animal-based proteins to cater for diverse dietary choices and nutritional demands.

4. Healthy Fats: Don't forget to add healthy fats to your grain bowl to boost taste, texture, and satiety. Add items like avocado slices, crumbled goat cheese or feta, roasted nuts or seeds (like sesame, pumpkin, or walnuts), or a drizzle of olive oil for a dose of heart-healthy lipids.

5. Tasty Dressings and Sauces: To enhance the flavors in your grain bowl, use dressings or sauces that mix well together. For convenience, use store-bought versions of balsamic glaze, tahini dressing, peanut sauce, and lemon vinaigrette, or try crafting your own.

6. Texture Contrast: When assembling your grain bowl, take texture into mind for a delicious meal. Foods featuring a mix of crunchy, chewy, and creamy textures include crispy tofu, cooked grains, roasted almonds, and creamy avocado.

7. Customization Options: We invite readers to demonstrate their originality by personalizing their grain bowls to match their nutritional requirements and tastes. Give tips for altering or swapping ingredients to fit a range of dietary demands and preferences. Low-carb, dairy-free, and gluten-free grains are a few examples.

8. Meal Prep suggestions: Give suggestions on how to meal prep the ingredients for grain bowls in advance to save time and make it easy to eat healthier meals all week. Some suggestions include cutting veggies, marinating protein, making dressing or sauce components ahead of time, and preparing cereals.

Quick and Nutritious Soups

A simple and pleasant alternative on hectic days when you need a filling meal quickly are quick and wholesome soups. These delectable soups, which may be eaten as a pleasant snack, a light lunch, or a hot supper, are rich with vitamins and minerals that will elevate your mood and feed your body. Here's how to generate appealing material about fast and wholesome soups:

1. easy Ingredients: Stress how easy and fast soups are to cook; most only require a few basic ingredients that you most likely already have on hand. Start with a tasty foundation, such as canned tomatoes or broth, and then top with veggies, protein, grains, or legumes for a substantial and fulfilling meal.

2. Easy Preparation: Emphasize how easy and quick soup preparation is, making it great for busy weeknights or days. Many soups may be cooked in 30 minutes or less, so you may enjoy a tasty supper without spending hours in the kitchen.

3. Variable Options: Emphasize how soups may be adjusted to fit taste preferences, dietary restrictions, and ingredient availability. Whether you enjoy creamy pureed soups, substantial chunky soups, or light broths, there's a soup recipe for every taste and scenario.

4. Nutrient-Rich Ingredients: Highlight the advantages of the foods that are typically used in satisfying and fast soups. Vegetables like carrots, celery, onions, and leafy greens are wonderful sources of important vitamins and minerals; protein sources like chicken, tofu, beans, and lentils are good sources of satiating protein and fiber.

5. Flavorful Enhancements: Showcase how easy it is to add flavor to soups by utilizing aromatics, spices, and ordinary herbs. The flavor of soups may be enhanced without adding extra calories or salt by adding pantry staples like garlic, ginger, and dry spices along with fresh herbs like parsley, cilantro, and basil.

6.Freezer-Friendly and Make-Ahead: Provide instructions on how to freeze soups for later use after they are made. Because the flavors have had time to blend, soups are a terrific meal prep alternative. They taste even better the following day. Freezer-safe containers make it simple to preserve individual quantities for fast and easy meals on busy days.

7. Balanced Nutrition: Emphasize how vital it is to cook soups with a reasonable ratio of healthy fats, carbs, and protein to keep you full and motivated. It is advised that readers add a variety of ingredients to their soups to ensure they are receiving a complete meal in each bowl.

8. Serving Suggestions: Serve soups with crusty bread, whole grain crackers, or a side salad to round out the meal and add extra fiber and minerals. Soups may also have toppings like grated cheese, chopped herbs, yogurt, or olive oil poured on top to increase taste and texture.

CHAPTER THREE

Delicious Meals

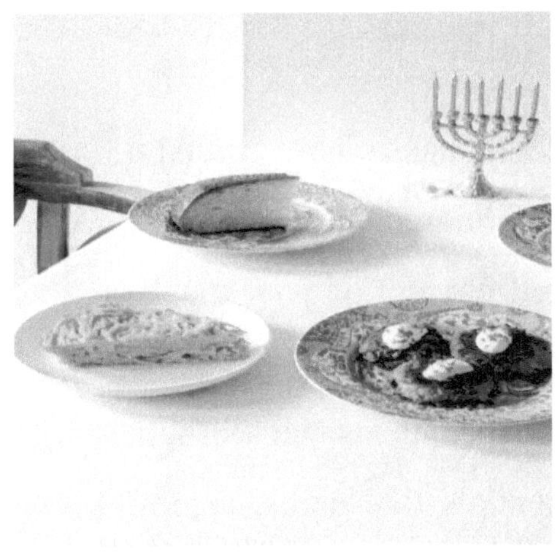

The finest way to conclude the day is to gather around the table with loved ones for a fantastic meal that fulfills both the body and the spirit. Whether you're cooking for one person, feeding the family, or hosting a dinner party, here's how to make intriguing content about excellent meals:

1. Inspirational dishes: Provide a range of delightful dinnertime alternatives that meet diverse dietary demands, palates, and culinary talents. Give ideas for simple and fast weekday dinners, comfortable classics,

daring and unexpected dishes, and special occasion desserts.

2. Fresh ingredients: Emphasize how crucial it is to utilize quality, fresh ingredients to improve the taste and nutritional content of your meals. Encourage readers to acquire seasonal vegetables, locally produced meats and seafood, as well as pantry essentials like herbs, spices, and nutritious grains, in order to make bright and delectable meals.

3. Well-Balanced Meals: Encourage meals that contain a decent mix of carbs and proteins, as well as a fair quantity of healthy fats, fruits, and vegetables. Give ideas for making balanced plates: half the plate should be made up of vegetables, 25% should be lean protein, and

25% should be made up of whole grains or starchy vegetables.

4. Creative cooking skills: Show off your inventive taste combinations and culinary abilities to raise your meals to the next level. If you want to give your food more taste and texture, consider roasting, grilling, braising, sautéing, and steaming. Encourage readers to try different cuisines and culinary techniques in order to widen their gourmet horizons.

5. Family-Friendly Options: Make meal ideas that will appeal to all members of the family, regardless of size. Give recipes for kid-friendly basics like homemade pizza, tacos with adjustable toppings, spaghetti and marinara sauce, and sheet pan meals that involve no cleaning.

6. Weekend Projects: Encourage readers to try more challenging recipes or to duplicate their favorite restaurant meals at home. This will transform making supper into a fun and creative weekend endeavor. Ideas for meals that may be made in advance and enjoyed throughout the week are welcomed.

7. Sharing and Community : Stress the social side of sharing wonderful meals with family and friends, whether you're throwing a potluck dinner party or just sitting down to a home-cooked meal. In order to develop lasting memories and form ties with family and friends, underline how much pleasure it is to cook and enjoy meals together.

8. Mindful Eating: Tell readers to slow down, appreciate each meal, and pay attention to their bodies' hunger and fullness signals throughout supper. Give advice on how to create a tranquil and comfortable eating atmosphere, including lowering the lights, playing relaxing music, and having a discussion with your dining mates.

Vegetarian food is incredibly tasty, healthy, versatile, and gratifying, indicating that plant-based meals can be just as full and satisfying as their meat-based counterparts. Whether you're a devout vegetarian or merely seeking to increase the amount of meatless meals in your diet, these vegetarian dishes are likely to delight even the pickiest eaters. This is how to make intriguing articles about fulfilling vegetarian recipes:

Satisfying Vegetarian Entrees

1.Creative Cuisine: When making vegetarian meals, encourage readers to explore diverse cuisines and taste profiles. There are lots of excellent vegetarian choices, from rich Mexican bean bowls and hot Indian curries to

Mediterranean-style chickpea salads and genuine Italian eggplant parmesan.

2. Whole Grains: Use whole grains to give vegetarian recipes additional texture, fiber, and nutrients. Grains include brown rice, quinoa, bulgur, farro, barley, and whole wheat pasta give a healthy basis for meals including salads, stir-fries, and bowls of grains.

3. Sauce and Seasoning: Emphasize the value of utilizing top-notch marinades, sauces, and spices to improve the flavor of vegetarian dishes. With the assistance of sauces and spices, basic meals may be transformed to exquisite nights. These might contain anything from tangy tomato sauces and creamy coconut curries to zesty herb dressings and scorching chili pastes.

4.Comfort Classics: Serve vegetarian versions on traditional comfort dishes to fulfill appetites for cozy tastes and textures. Vegetarian foods, such as mushroom risotto, black bean burgers, and lentil shepherd's pie, may be just as substantial and fulfilling as their meat-based equivalents.

5. Serve vegetarian dishes that may suit a large or small gathering of people Family Favorites. Creamy spinach and ricotta filled shells, heavy bean and vegetable stew, and veggie-loaded pasta primavera are guaranteed to satisfy even the pickiest palates.

6. Balanced Nutrition: Encourage readers to create vegetarian meals that are rich in a variety of proteins and carbs, as well as a decent number of fruits, vegetables, healthy fats, and other nutrients. By blending a range of nutrient-rich foods, vegetarian meals may incorporate all the components essential for a well-balanced diet.

Lean Protein Power Plates

For a tasty, healthful, and well-balanced lunch, power plates with lean protein are a fantastic alternative. These meals frequently contain a lean protein source as the main course and a range of nutrient-dense veggies, complete grains, and healthy fats as side dishes. Whether you want to gain muscle, decrease weight, or just feed your body nourishing nutrients, lean protein power plates are a pleasant and practical approach to satisfy your nutritional demands. Here's how to develop appealing material regarding lean protein-filled power plates:

1. **Protein Prowess**: Let me start by highlighting the function that lean protein plays in maintaining satiety, encouraging muscle

building, and assisting in weight control. Without swallowing an excessive number of calories or saturated fat, lean protein sources such as grilled chicken breast, turkey, fish, tofu, tempeh, lentils, and low-fat dairy products may supply high-quality protein.

2. Vibrant veggies: Emphasize the quantity of bright veggies that work well with lean protein on power platters. A variety of roasted, steamed, or leafy green vegetables, such as tomatoes, mushrooms, bell peppers, carrots, zucchini, and broccoli, may be included in your meal. Vegetables are a terrific source of vitamins, minerals, and antioxidants in addition to taste and texture.

3. Whole Grain Goodness: To give complex carbs, such as whole grains in power plates, that increase satiety and energy. Meals like quinoa, brown rice, barley, farro, bulgur, and whole wheat pasta or bread may all contain fiber, protein, and vital minerals. Choose whole grains over processed grains for the maximum nutritional advantages.

4. Healthy Fats: Don't forget to incorporate healthy fats on lean protein power plates to boost taste, texture, and satiety. To receive your portion of heart-healthy monounsaturated fats, sprinkle some nuts, seeds, avocado slices, or olive oil over your meal. Fatty fish like salmon and trout may also be excellent sources of omega-3 fatty acids.

5. Flavorful Seasonings: Experiment with different herbs, spices, and marinades to add some flavor and variation to your lean protein power plates. Try adding herbs like thyme, rosemary, and oregano to chicken, marinating tofu in a sour soy-ginger sauce, or flavoring fish

CHAPTER FOUR

healthy snack

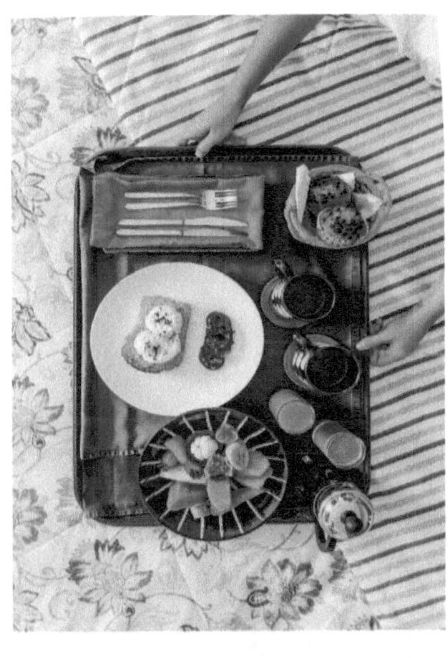

with a spicy citrus rub. Try experimenting with different taste combinations without fear.

6. Customization Options: Provide options for customizing power plates depending on dietary restrictions, personal preferences, and nutritional objectives. Offer low-carb, gluten-free, or vegetarian alternatives to fit varied dietary demands and lifestyles.

Eating nutrient-dense snacks helps with energy maintenance, general health enhancement, and appetite control between meals. They allow your body a chance to absorb the vital nutrients it needs, fulfill cravings, and avoid overindulging later in the day. Here's how to make intriguing articles about nutritious snacks:

1. Nutrient Density: Snacks that are rich in vitamins, minerals, and other essential nutrients compared to their calorie count are advised for readers to pick. Various foods such as fruits, vegetables, nuts, seeds, and whole grains offer a diversity of nutrients that improve general well-being.

2. Balanced Macronutrients: Promote satiety and sustained energy by distributing protein, carbs, and healthy fats in a balanced way in snacks. Combining these macronutrients decreases hunger and stabilizes blood sugar levels. One may produce a nice nutritious combination, for example, by combining almond butter with apple slices or cheese with whole grain crackers.

3. Portion Control: Emphasize the need of reducing your snacking portion sizes in order to avoid eating excessive quantities of calories. Encourage readers to think about portion proportions and to abstain from mindlessly swallowing food right out of the packaging. Preparing meals in tiny quantities in advance could help avoid overindulgence.

4. Hydration: Readers should be encouraged to remain hydrated during the day as sometimes, thirst and hunger could be confused for one another. It's advisable to eat snacks in addition to a glass of water to keep hydrated and feel full.

5.healthy Foods: Encourage the consumption of healthy foods instead of processed snacks whenever feasible. In order to maintain their natural nutrients, fiber, and antioxidants, whole foods require minimum processing. Encourage readers to pick fresh fruits and vegetables combined with whole foods, nuts, and seeds to prepare whole-food snacks at home.

6. Convenience: Provide options for lightweight, simply reachable snacks that are suited for consuming while on the move. Whole fruit, trail mix, individual amounts of Greek yogurt, and precut veggies with hummus are simple and fast solutions for individuals with hectic schedules.

7. range: Readers are recommended to diversify their snacks to ensure they acquire a range of nutrients and to minimize boredom. Offer suggestions for salty, sweet, crunchy, creamy, and creamy snacks to satisfy a range of palates.

8. Homemade Options: Inspire readers to whip up some healthful, homemade snacks in the kitchen by utilizing their imagination. Recipes for items like yogurt parfaits, energy balls, veggie chips, and homemade granola bars enable you to manage and change the components.

Homemade trail mixes are a nutritious and varied snack choice that offer a simple and quick method to provide your body the nutrients it needs to improve your energy levels while you're out and about. Trail mixes are a great blend of tastes, textures, and nutrients that will sustain you during a rigorous job, on the trails, or to satisfy your hunger after a workout. This is how to generate compelling material about producing your own trail mix:

Homemade Trail Mixes

1. Nutrient-Rich products: emphasizes the diversity of nutrient-rich goods that may be utilized to produce trail mixes. A few nuts and seeds that may be used as a basis are cashews, almonds, peanuts, walnuts, pumpkin seeds, and sunflower seeds. These foods offer necessary vitamins and minerals, protein, and healthy fats.

2. Dried Fruits: add dried fruits to trail mixes to naturally sweeten, chew, and deliver a blast of flavor. Natural sugars, which are contained in foods like cranberries, mangoes, apricots, cherries, and raisins, supply you with rapid energy and are also rich in fiber, vitamins, and minerals.

3. Whole Grains: Add whole grains, such as granola, popcorn, pretzels, or whole grain cereal, to trail mixes to give them crunch, texture, and extra fiber. Select whole grain foods with less added sugar for prolonged energy and fullness.

4. Sweet and Savory Additions: Try blending sweet and savory ingredients to build unique and delightful trail mixes. Additions such as dark chocolate chips, yogurt-covered raisins, coconut flakes, dried edamame, or roasted chickpeas may fulfill desires for both sweet and salty sensations.

5. Spices and Seasonings: To improve the taste of your homemade trail mixes, add a variety of spices and seasonings. Consider adding a dab of pumpkin spice, nutmeg, or cinnamon for added warmth and flavor. Combine some savory spices, such as onion, garlic, or chili powder, with nuts and seeds for a fiery explosion.

6. Customization Options: We invite readers to modify their trail mixes to fit their own nutritional choices, inclinations, and energy requirements. Provide recommendations for incorporating additional components such as hemp hearts, protein powder, dried herbs, or even a tiny dose of sea salt to make a customized mix that meets their own tastes.

7. Portion Control: Trail mix makes a nice snack, but it's easy to overeat because it tastes so delicious and is so handy. Remind readers to control their portion quantities at all times. It is advisable to portion trail mix in advance and store it in tiny bags or containers to assist avoid mindless nibbling and maintain optimal quantity levels.

8. Storage and Shelf Life: Provide tips on how to keep homemade trail mixes fresher longer. Trail mixes should be kept in sealed containers or resealable bags in a cool, dry area away from direct sunlight. When kept carefully, trail mix may last for several weeks, making it a helpful snack for individuals with hectic schedules.

Tasty and Nutritious Spreads and Dips

Nutritious and tasty spreads and dips may serve as an adaptable base for a range of cuisines, offering extra nutrition, taste, and texture. If you're searching for a fast and simple snack, preparing a packed lunch, or entertaining guests, these spreads and dips give a ton of inventive and delightful possibilities. Here's how to develop fascinating content about healthy, tasty spreads and dips:

1 Fresh products: Emphasize the significance of producing tasty and wholesome spreads and dips with excellent, newly purchased products. Add a variety of fresh herbs,

vegetables, fruits, and nuts to your cuisine to give it bright color, delectable flavor, and necessary nutrients.

2. Protein-Rich Bases: Start with protein-rich alternatives such as Greek yogurt, hummus, tahini, cottage cheese, or white beans to create a tasty and nutritional basis for your dips and spreads. These components not only give richness and creaminess, but they also provide critical vitamins and amino acids that promote overall well being.

3. Flavorful Enhancements: Experiment with different herbs, spices, and condiments to improve the taste of your spreads and dips. You may add components like garlic, lemon juice, cumin, paprika, chili powder, or fresh basil to create flavor combinations that are unique and agreeable to your taste.

4. Texture Variations: Offer a selection of textures to satisfy diverse demands and tastes. Blend ingredients until smooth for creamy dips or spreads, or leave them slightly chunky for texture and visual appeal. Add-ins like chopped nuts, seeds, or dried fruits may give some crunch and visual appeal.

5. Vegetable-Based selections: Highlight the diversity of vegetable-based spreads and dips, which give a delightful and wholesome alternative for conventional selections. Nutritious vegetable-based recipes include roasted red pepper hummus, avocado salsa, beet and walnut dip, and spinach and artichoke dip.

6. Whole Grain Dippers: Whole wheat tortilla chips, sliced veggies, whole wheat pita bread, or whole grain crackers may be used as dippers or spreads. The complex carbs, fiber, vitamins, and minerals present in whole grains assist to increase sensations of enjoyment and fullness.

7. Healthier Substitutions: To minimize calories, added sugars, and saturated fats without compromising taste or texture, substitute out conventional components with healthier ones. Replace butter in spreads with avocado, Greek yogurt in creamy dips in lieu of mayonnaise, and sugary spreads in favor of unsweetened nut butter.

8. Serving recommendations: offer recommendations on how to offer spreads and dips other than the usual dipping situation. Spread them on toast or crackers, sprinkle them into salads or grain bowls, use them as a delicious topping for grilled meats or veggies, or use them as a filler in sandwiches or wraps.

CHAPTER

FIVE

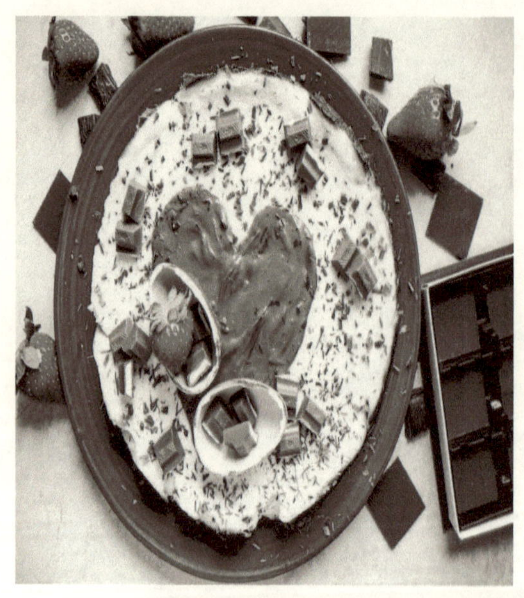

Candy Goods

Sweet foods are a beautiful pleasure that brighten every day and satisfy wishes. Sweet sweets are delightful and helpful in many ways, despite their usual connection with sugary pastries and opulent delights. Here's how to create compelling stuff about desserts:

1. Natural Sweeteners: When cooking sweet sweets, advise readers to use natural sweeteners like dates, honey, or maple syrup. Compared to refined sugar, these replacements give sweetness mixed with added minerals and antioxidants, making them healthier choices.

2. Whole Food Ingredients: Emphasize how adding whole foods to sweet treats may boost their healthy value. Incorporate fiber, protein, healthy fats, vitamins, and other nutrients into your meals by utilizing foods like oats, nuts, seeds, fruits, and dark chocolate.

3. Balanced Recipes: To induce satiety and prevent blood sugar spikes, support the manufacture of sweet sweets that deliver a balance of macronutrients. Incorporate healthy fats and protein sources with your carbohydrates to help slow down the speed at which sugar enters your system.

4. Mindful Eating: When indulging in sweets, urge readers to eat consciously by slowing down, enjoying each bite, and being aware of their body's signals of hunger and fullness. To truly experience the flavors and textures of sweet delicacies, it is essential to eat them in a tranquil and comfortable situation.

5. Fruit-Based sweets: Emphasize the intrinsic sweetness and health benefits of sweets produced with fruit. Provide fruit salad, skewer, baked crisp, and frozen fruit popsicle meals that accentuate the flavors and textures present in fresh fruit.

6. Healthier Baking Techniques: Give tips on how to bake in a manner that utilizes less added sugar and fat. Some suggestions are to use whole wheat flour or almond flour for increased fiber, bake with applesauce or ripe bananas for natural sweetness, and use less butter or added oils in recipes.

7. Creative Twists: Encourage readers to use their ideas in the kitchen to create creative flavor combinations and switch out items for tasty surprises. To give their creations greater depth and complexity, encourage them to venture beyond the box and experiment with unusual ingredients like matcha, coconut, spices, or herbs.

Rich But Nutritious Desserts

Desserts that blend pleasure and healthfulness deliver the best of both worlds: the delight of a rich dessert without compromising critical nutrients. Healthy ingredients, natural sweeteners, and imaginative flavor combinations are utilized to produce these treats, which will quench cravings and boost overall health and wellness. Here's how to create compelling articles about rich but wholesome desserts:

1. Nutrient-Dense Additions: To boost the nutritional value of desserts, use nutrient-dense add-ins like nuts or seeds, dried fruits, and dark chocolate chips. Fiber, protein, and beneficial fats from these foods help to control blood sugar levels and increase fullness.

2. Lower Sugar Content: Provide recipes for delectable treats that are healthful without losing taste by using less sugar or other sweeteners. To reach sweetness without the downsides of refined sugar, consider experimenting with natural sweeteners like stevia, monk fruit, or coconut sugar.

3. Portion regulation: To prevent overindulging and limit calorie intake, advocate portion control while relishing delicious treats. To aid lessen portion sizes while still meeting demands, propose creating mini-sized sweets or presenting desserts in smaller amounts.

4. Balanced Macronutrients: Include healthy fats and sources of protein in addition to carbohydrates to create a balance of macronutrients in rich sweets. This fosters persistent satiety by slowing the bloodstream's absorption of sugar.

5. Healthier Baking procedures: Provide advice on baking procedures that eliminate the need for additional fats and oils. Part recommendations are to limit the number of added sugars in recipes, use mashed avocado or banana instead of butter, and substitute part of the flour with oat flour or almond flour for additional fiber.

6. Creative Flavor Combinations: Encourage readers to experiment with diverse ingredient pairings and flavor combinations to improve the flavor of sumptuous treats. Try altering the spices, herbs, extracts, and natural flavorings to give desserts more complexity and richness without increasing the quantity of calories or sugar.

7. Mindful Enjoyment: When indulging in sumptuous sweets, urge readers to practice mindful eating by slowing down, enjoying each mouthful, and being aware of their body's signals of hunger and fullness. Encourage moderation in dessert intake as a component of a healthy diet and way of life.

Fruit-Sided Treats

Fruit-focused sweets are a pleasant and wholesome way to indulge in the natural flavors and healthiness of fresh fruits while fulfilling your sweet desire. These treats, which may be eaten as a light dessert, a refreshing snack, or a vivid side dish, are rich with vitamins, minerals, fiber, and antioxidants that improve overall health and wellness. Here's how to create captivating content about luscious fruit:

1. Options Packed with Nutrients: Stress the health benefits of adding fruits to sweets and snacks. Fruits are abundant in critical vitamins and minerals like vitamin C, potassium, and folate while naturally low in calories and fat. Additionally, they have dietary fiber, which assists in digestion and keeps you feeling satisfied and full.

2. simple and Adaptable meals: Provide simple and adaptable recipes that accentuate the innate flavors and sweetness of fruits. There are various ways to make wonderful fruit-focused snacks that fit a range of tastes and preferences, from fruit salads and parfaits to smoothie bowls and fruit kabobs.

3. Creative combinations: When mixing fruits into sweets and snacks, readers are encouraged to experiment with new flavor combinations. Try adding yogurt, nuts, seeds, honey, cinnamon, and mint, or other complimenting ingredients to enhance the taste and texture of fruit-focused treats.

4.better Dessert Options: Offer fruit-focused desserts as a better option for conventional sweets that are high in fat and added sugar. Fruit-based sweets are a guilt-free solution for individuals who wish to enjoy healthily as they may sate sweet cravings without the need for extra sugar or useless calories.

5. Seasonal Inspiration: Stress how vital it is to employ seasonal fruits in fruit-focused desserts in order to benefit from their finest quality, affordability, and freshness. To take advantage of the greatest that each season has to offer, urge readers to go to their local farmers' markets or choose their own fruits at orchards.

6. Entertaining and Kid-Friendly Creations: Offer recommendations for entertaining and kid-friendly fruit-focused delights that will make fruit eating joyful for the entire family. In order to excite children's senses and tempt them to try new fruits and flavors, be creative with fruit shapes, colors, and presentations.

Delightful and Airy Bakings

Beautiful and light baked items are the right blend of pleasure and healthfulness, offering you a guilt-free chance to satisfy your sweet desire without compromising the nutrients that your body needs. These baked products are a perfect compliment to any gathering because of their nutrient-rich components, light texture, and delicate flavors. This is how to create compelling content about airy and tasty baked goods:

1. Healthy Ingredients: To improve nutritional value, emphasize the use of healthy, premium ingredients in airy, elegant baked items. To add extra fiber and minerals, look for whole grains like almond flour, oats, or whole wheat flour. To cut down on processed sugar, select natural sweeteners like dates, honey, or maple syrup.

2. Reduced Fat Content: Provide recipes for baked items that contain less fat to make them lighter and lower in calories and saturated fat. Use ingredients such as avocado, mashed bananas, applesauce, Greek yogurt, or mashed bananas to offer richness and moisture without using too much butter or oil.

3. Adding Fruits and vegetables: Highlight how versatile fruits and veggies are by adding them into airy and elegant baked products. Grated carrots or zucchini may offer structure and moisture to muffins or bread; berries, apples, or citrus fruits may provide natural sweetness and flavor to cakes, scones, or tarts.

5. Healthier Baking Methods: Give tips on how to bake in a healthier manner by using less added sugar and fat. Some recommendations are to use nonstick cooking spray rather than butter or oil to coat pans, cut down on sugar in dishes, and add fruits and vegetables for natural sweetness and moisture.

6. Gluten-Free and Vegan Options: Provide light and attractive baked products that are both gluten-free and vegan in order to satisfy a range of dietary preferences and limits. Try gluten-free options such as rice flour, quinoa flour, or coconut flour, and for vegan recipes, use plant-based ingredients such as flaxseed meal, chia seeds, or aquafaba in lieu of eggs.

Fit and flavorful

CHAPTER SIX

Lifestyle Suggestions

A wide array of habits and routines that

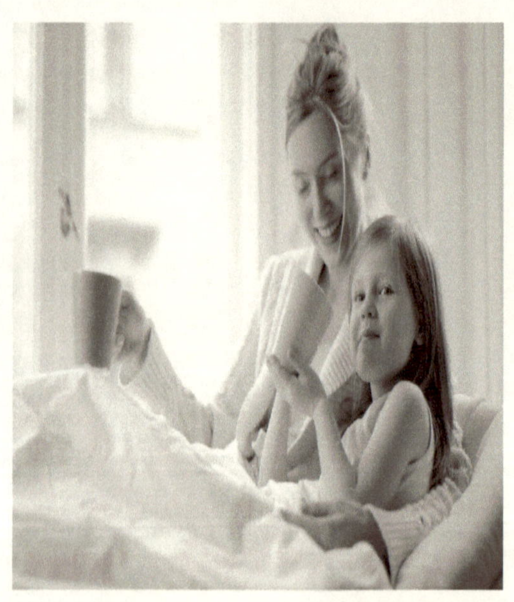

improve overall health, happiness, and well-being are covered in lifestyle advice. These advice span a broad variety of themes, such as relationships, work-life balance, mental and physical health, and personal development. People may acquire a sense of satisfaction and pleasure and enhance their quality of life by incorporating excellent lifestyle habits into their regular activities. Consider these crucial lifestyle suggestions:

1. Make Physical Activity a Priority: Find activities you enjoy doing and fit them into your daily routine to make regular exercise a priority. Most days of the week, strive to get in at least 30 minutes of moderate-intensity exercise to build flexibility, strength, and cardiovascular health.

2. Nourish Your Body: Make sure you consume a diet rich in whole grains, fruits, vegetables, lean meats, healthy fats, and a balance of nutrients. Drink lots of water to keep hydrated throughout the day, and cut down on processed foods, sugar-filled drinks, and too much alcohol.

3. Practice attention: Use practices like yoga, deep breathing exercises, or meditation to increase present-moment awareness and attention. These strategies may benefit in decreasing stress, boosting attention and concentration, and developing emotional wellness.

4. Acquire Sufficient Sleep: Make sleep a priority and build a regular sleep routine to assure you obtain the required 7-9 hours of restful sleep every night. To support restful sleep, develop a peaceful nightly routine, restrict screen time before bed, and give a warm resting place.

5. Nurture Relationships: Devote time and effort to building and keeping strong relationships with loved ones, family, and friends. Schedule regular social time, express your appreciation and admiration, and be honest and transparent in your communication.

6. Manage Stress: To properly manage stress and prevent burnout, use healthy coping mechanisms. To aid lessen feelings of overburden and worry, participate in stress-reduction methods like mindfulness, deep breathing, physical activity, and time management.

7. Find Work-Life Balance: Make an effort to maintain your personal life, work, and leisure activities in a healthy balance. Establish limitations on employment duties, give self-care and downtime top priority, and arrange leisure time for interests, hobbies, and relaxation.

8. continual Education and Development: Adopt a growth attitude and grab possibilities for continual education and self-improvement.

Establish targets, explore new interests, challenge yourself to go beyond your comfort zone, and appreciate your success along the way.

9.Practice Gratitude: Develop a thankful mentality by continuously identifying and appreciating the wonderful things in your life. Express your thanks for the people and events in your life, write in a gratitude notebook, and focus on the positives you have rather than what you need.

10. Seek Support When Needed: If you're experiencing problems with mental health concerns, stress, or life changes, don't be reluctant to seek support from trustworthy friends, family members, or specialists. Seeking aid from others is a sign of strength, and support networks may give insightful guidance, inspiration, and perspective.

Conscientious Purchasing and Menu Planning

To save time, prevent food waste, and maintain a healthful diet, it's necessary to plan your meals and shop intelligently. By utilizing these strategies, consumers may save money, cook meals more efficiently during the week, and make informed choices about what they purchase. Here's how to generate compelling information about meal planning and prudent shopping:

1. **Make a shopping List:** Start by writing the required pantry supplies and the meals you have planned for the following week on your shopping list. Make a list of the products you need to purchase and take stock of what you already have by checking through your pantry, freezer, and refrigerator. To make your shopping

trip more effective, compose your list according to dietary categories.

2. Plan Meals in Advance: Set aside some time to arrange your meals, including breakfast, lunch, dinner, and snacks, for the upcoming week. When picking meals, take into consideration aspects like dietary preferences, nutritional aims, and time restrictions. To assure balanced nutrition, strive to eat the proper quantity of protein, carbohydrates, and healthy fats at each meal.

3. Shop with Purpose: Refrain from making impulsive purchases and stick to your shopping list when you shop at the farmers' market or grocery store. Pay attention to reductions and discounts on nutritious staples like fruits, vegetables, lean meats, and whole grains, but resist the impulse to acquire needless products.

4. Select Seasonal and Local food: Whenever practicable, pick seasonal and locally produced food over out-of-season or imported choices as it's generally fresher, tastier, and less costly. In addition to assisting area farmers, seasonal food lowers its influence on the environment by needing fewer trip kilometers.

5. Research Labels: To make informed judgments about the things you're purchasing, take the time to study ingredient lists and food labels. Prioritize natural foods with recognizable components and hunt for those with the fewest added sugars, salt, and artificial additives.

6. Buy in Bulk and Batch Cook: When buying non-perishables like grains, legumes, nuts, and seeds in big amounts, you may save money and time. Ensuring you always have nutritional choices accessible and simplifying meal preparation during the week may be done by batch cooking significant quantities of grains, meats, and vegetables on weekends.

7. Minimize Food Waste: Plan meals that make use of perishable ingredients before they go bad to help cut down on food waste. Make fresh dishes with leftover meats, vegetables, or grains, or add them to salads, soups, or stir-fries. For subsequent meals, keep leftovers in the freezer or refrigerator in sealed containers.

8. Stay Adaptable: Adjust your shopping list and meal plan to fit your requirements and preferences as well as availability and sales. Never hesitate to replace or alter as required to allow for unanticipated situations or schedule adjustments.

9.advantage Technology to Your Advantage: To make grocery shopping and meal planning simpler, make advantage of digital coupons, online grocery delivery services, and meal planning programs. You can make smarter food purchases, save time, and keep order with the assistance of these tools.

10. Review and Adjust: After completing your weekly meal plan and shopping, take some time to review your progress and make any required improvements to your approach. **To** make the most of your shopping and meal planning routine, review what went well and what may be done better. Then, make the required modifications.

Practices of Mindful Eating

Eating and drinking thoughtfully means devoting your total attention to the activity, both within and outside. It requires being attentive to the flavors, textures, and sensations of food in addition to the emotions, thoughts, and body signals associated with eating. People may create a stronger relationship with food, enjoy meals more, and feel better overall by participating in mindful eating activities. You should add the following crucial mindful eating practices into your normal routine:

1. Eat attentively and Chew Thoroughly: Take your time, chewing every mouthful entirely before swallowing. Eat each meal carefully and thoughtfully. This supports enhanced digestion by more completely breaking down food and letting you appreciate the flavors and textures of your meal to the fullest.

2. Engage All Five Senses: During eating, pay attention to the tastes, textures, sounds, colors, and fragrances of your food. Observe how your meal appears, how the components smell, how it sounds as you chew, and how your taste buds respond to the flavor.

3. Pay Attention to Your Body's Cues About Hunger and Fullness: Use these cues to help you make smart eating choices. Rather than eating because you're bored, anxious, or merely out of habit, eat when you're physically hungry and stop when you're full. Throughout meals, take periodic intervals to monitor your levels of hunger and fullness.

4. Remove Distractions: By switching off the TV, putting away devices, and focusing simply on the activity of eating, you may eliminate distractions while you're eating. This keeps you from overindulging in food without thinking and helps you to be more attentive of it.

5. Cultivate Gratitude: Show thanks for the people and resources that went into creating the food on your plate. Give some attention to how your food goes from the farm to your plate and express thanks for the nourishment it supplies.

6. careful Portion Control: Be careful of serving sizes and judge how much food is good for you based on your degree of hunger and nutritional needs. To aid limit portion sizes and prevent overindulging, use smaller bowls and plates. Also, try not to return for seconds unless you are truly hungry.

7. Be Non-Judgmental: Take a non-judgmental attitude to eating, abstaining from labeling foods as "good" or "bad." Give yourself freedom to enjoy any food in moderation and guilt-free, stressing variety, balance, and general nourishment.

8. Engage in Mindful Snacking: Choose healthful foods and relish them in the present by employing mindful eating approaches to your snacking. Take your time to savor and enjoy every bite of your meal rather than nibbling away mindlessly while engaged.

9. Listen to Your Body: Observe your physical, mental, and emotional reactions to varied meals. After ingesting a given meal, pay attention to any physiological reactions or sensations and alter your diet to meet your body's individual needs and preferences.

10. Reflect on Your Eating Habits: Without passing judgment, evaluate your eating habits, views about food, and emotions associated with it. Take notice of any habits or patterns you may have, and think about how you may build a more attentive and nutritious eating approach.

Maintaining Your Motivation and Activity

Maintaining physical health, mental clarity, and overall energy involves staying engaged and motivated. Finding techniques to sustain your desire and devotion to frequent physical activity may be tough at times, regardless of your degree of expertise with exercise. However, you can construct a fitness plan that will stay and keep you feeling and moving your best provided you have the necessary skills and approach. Here are some crucial ideas to help you keep motivated and active:

1. Set Realistic Goals: Make sure your fitness targets are sensible, achievable, and in accordance with your priorities, interests, and talents. Whether your purpose is to decrease weight, raise your overall fitness level, or run a marathon, breaking it down into smaller, more manageable objectives will help you keep motivated and focused as you go.

2. Find Activities You adore: Try out a range of physical pastimes to determine which ones you actually love and excitedly anticipate indulging in. Selecting activities that you enjoy and find rewarding, such as dancing, swimming, cycling, hiking, or team sports, can help you stay motivated and devoted to regular exercise.

3. Create a Consistent Routine: Plan frequent workouts into your daily or weekly agenda to develop a consistent fitness plan. Exercise should be treated like any other big commitment; regard it as a non-negotiable appointment with yourself.

4. Mix It Up: Add diversity to your routine to keep your workouts interesting and exciting. To keep things exciting and original, try various exercise routines, mix up your training area, and take part in group fitness classes or challenges.

5. Create Incentives and Rewards: Reward yourself when you reach fitness targets and maintain consistency in your training plan. Offering yourself a reward for a job well done, such as a new exercise apparel, a massage or spa day, or a healthy snack after your workout, can help you keep motivated and goal-focused.

6. Find an Accountability or Workout Partner: Having a friend, family member, or workout partner as a partner may assist to raise motivation, give accountability, and support. exercise may be more enjoyable when you train with someone, and it may also help you keep on track when things go difficult.

7. Track Your success: To stay motivated and assess your success, maintain a diary of your workouts, successes, and progress. Tracking your progress, whether via a spreadsheet, notepad, or fitness app, may drive you to keep trying new activities and give you a sense of success.

8. Stay Positive and Flexible: Remain cheery and self-compassionate, especially in the face of setbacks or times of low motivation. Recall that progress is not always straight-line, and experiencing ups and downs is natural. To get beyond hurdles and continue on course, be adaptive and flexible in your approach.

9. Pay Attention to How You Feel: Observe your physiological and mental condition after working out. Regular physical activity provides you a boost in confidence, energy, and attitude. Take advantage of these wonderful feelings to keep pushing yourself forward.

10. Celebrate Your Successes: Acknowledge the work and dedication it needs to attain your objectives, no matter how small. Marking victories, attaining targets, and defeating barriers boosts your will to sustain your long-term drive and activity.

CONCLUSION

In summation, expecting a healthy future is an exhilarating journey full of opportunity, promise, and endless growth opportunities. It's a journey that begins with a choice to put our health and wellbeing first and continues on with modest, achievable acts in the direction of change.

Looking ahead, we envision ourselves having busy, gratifying lives that are overflowing with life and vitality. We imagine ourselves adopting more health-conscious practices, feeding our body good foods, and obtaining regular exercise that boosts our overall welfare.

Anticipating the future, we find inspiration in the concept of being more competent, resilient, and strong enough to confront life's problems.

As we build a stronger connection with ourselves and the world around us, we feel ourselves radiating self-assurance, contentment, and inner tranquility.

But there are hurdles along the route to a healthy future. We might encounter hurdles, temptations, and periods of doubt along the path. However, it is because of these trials that we recognize our own strength and tenacity. We develop the capacity to modify, endure, and retain our focus on our goals in the face of difficulties.

Let us bear in mind that progress is not always linear as we begin out on our adventure. There will be triumphs and disappointments, ups and downs. But we are getting closer to our goal of health and wellness with every step we take.

Anticipating a healthy future implies embracing the path, its progress, and its change in addition to the eventual aim. Honoring our body and ourselves entails making choices that are congruent with our aims and values.

Thus, let us proceed on this voyage with open minds and hearts. Let's delight in our achievements, learn lessons from our mistakes, and keep forging forward with courage and persistence. Together, we can design a future that exceeds our greatest expectations in terms of brightness, health, and vitality.

Honoring your health journey serves as a poignant reminder of the gains you've made, the hurdles you've overcome, and the devotion you've shown to putting your health first. Maintaining motivation, improving self-confidence, and maintaining long-term progress all rely on taking the time to acknowledge and celebrate your successes, whether you've achieved a key milestone, fulfilled a specific goal, or simply continued to put in steady effort.

In your search for health and wellness, you may generate a deeper sense of fulfillment and joy by adopting an attitude of gratitude, self-compassion, and appreciation for the path. Honoring the daily choices, habits, and acts that boost your overall welfare and quality of life is just as vital as celebrating your health journey's arrival.

Thus, stop to celebrate your progress, acknowledge your victories, and repeat your determination to lead a successful and healthy life. Discover techniques to honor your health journey and greet the path ahead with optimism, resilience, and a sense of pride in everything that you've done. This may be done in a multitude of ways, such as by a modest act of self-care, a sincere statement of gratitude, or a happy celebration with loved ones. In order to become the happiest and healthiest version of yourself, never forget that every success, no matter how tiny, is grounds for celebration.